Copyright © 2022 by Linda Caroline

All rights reserved. No part of this publication may be reproduced, distributed, or transmitted in any form or by any means, including photocopying, recording, or other electronic or mechanical methods, without the prior written permission of the publisher, except in the case of brief quotation embodied in critical reviews and certian other noncommercial uses permitted by copyright law.

## Table of Contents

Introduction ............................................................................ 3

What is LPR? ........................................................................... 5

Symptoms ............................................................................... 7

Causes .................................................................................... 11

Diagnosis ................................................................................ 13

Treatment .............................................................................. 15

Complications ........................................................................ 18

Which foods should I eat or avoid if I have silent reflux? ......... 20

Natural and home remedies .................................................... 34

Recipes for LPR ...................................................................... 45

Conclusion ............................................................................. 91

## Introduction

If you've ever overdone it on pizza and beer, you may be familiar with the discomfort of acid reflux. Heartburn, chest pain, and nausea are all hallmarks of reflux.

The symptoms are unmistakable. But for some people, the symptoms of reflux aren't so obvious. In fact, they're silent.

Laryngopharyngeal reflux (LPR) is also known as silent reflux. LPR doesn't cause any symptoms. The contents of your stomach could reflux up your esophagus, into your throat and voice box, and even into your nasal passages, and you might never know it — until more serious symptoms begin to arise from damage caused by stomach acid.

Laryngopharyngeal reflux is a condition in which acid that is made in the stomach travels up the esophagus (swallowing tube) and gets to the throat. Symptoms include sore throat and an irritated larynx (voice box). Treatments consist mostly of lifestyle changes.

## What is LPR?

Laryngopharyngeal reflux is a condition in which acid from the stomach travels up the esophagus through a relaxed lower esophageal sphincter (LES) and into throat. The LES controls the opening between the esophagus and the stomach, which should remain closed tightly except when you're swallowing food.

Laryngopharyngeal reflux affects many people each year, many of whom have no clue…so how do you know if you have it? LPR, as it's also called, is often hard to spot because of its lack of present symptoms or symptoms that coincide with other diseases, such as GERD.

When the upper esophageal sphincter doesn't function properly, the acid that has back flowed into the esophagus enters the throat and voice box. When this happens, it's called laryngopharyngeal reflux, or LPR.[1]

Although they are each caused by a malfunction of esophageal sphincters, LPR is not the same thing as heartburn. Heartburn occurs when the lower (rather than the upper) esophageal sphincter malfunctions. In addition, LPR symptoms are concentrated in the throat and voice box, while heartburn is felt more in the chest.

## Symptoms

The symptoms of silent reflux in infants and children include:

- coughing
- vomiting
- failure to grow and gain weight
- asthma
- a sore throat
- hoarseness
- noisy breathing
- ear infections
- feeding difficulties
- turning blue
- aspiration, or inhaling food and other particles into the lungs

It is common for infants to spit up, but problems with breathing and feeding could be signs of a more serious health problem. A doctor should investigate these symptoms.

Children with silent reflux will not always vomit or regurgitate.

Researchers are currently exploring possible links between silent reflux in children and recurrent ear infections and sinusitis.

Some symptoms, such as projectile vomiting or vomit that contains blood, could be indications of other health problems. Visit a health professional if these symptoms become evident.

When acid reflux leads to persistent heartburn, occurring maybe twice a week for 3 weeks or more, this is known as gastroesophageal reflux disease, or GERD. Silent reflux, or laryngeal-pharyngeal reflux (LPR), is similar, but without the heartburn and indigestion.

**Other Symptoms**

When acid passes quickly through the esophagus but pools in the throat, you may experience LPR symptoms. These symptoms are concentrated in your throat and voice box and include:
- Continual throat clearing
- Chronic throat irritation
- Chronic cough
- Hoarseness
- Excessive phlegm in the throat
- Dysphagia (difficulty swallowing)
- Constant sensation of something in the throat
- Consumed food comes back up
- Postnasal drainage

- Weak voice
- Cracking voice
- Blockage of the breathing passage
- Spasm of the larynx (voice box)
- Wheezing

People with LPR don't typically experience classic heartburn symptoms (unless, of course, they also have gastroesophageal reflux disease or GERD). That's because, for refluxed acid to cause heartburn, it has to stay in the esophagus long enough to irritate. With LPR, acid usually passes quickly through the esophagus.

## Causes

There are two sphincter muscles located in the esophagus. When either malfunction they result in different conditions and symptoms:

Lower esophageal sphincter (LES): When the lower esophageal sphincter is not functioning correctly, it backflows stomach acid into the esophagus. This backflow causes acid reflux and chest pain. If this happens two or more times a week, it can be a sign of GERD.2

Upper esophageal sphincter (UES): When the upper esophageal sphincter doesn't function correctly, acid enters the throat, where it pools and irritates the throat and voice box.

LPR occurs when the UES malfunctions and acid pools in the throat.

## Diagnosis

To diagnose LPR, your healthcare provider will do a physical exam and take a medical history. Often, doctors do not need to order tests to make a diagnosis. However, they may do one of the following tests to determine if you have LPR:

- Swallowing test: In this test, you swallow a liquid that coats the esophagus, stomach, and intestines so your doctor can see them on an X-ray.
- Laryngoscopy: This procedure allows your doctor to see changes in the throat and voice box.
- 24-hour pH testing: If too much stomach acid moves into the upper esophagus or throat, this procedure may help your doctor see what's going on. This test uses two pH sensors—one at

the bottom of the esophagus and one at the top. These sensors will let the healthcare provider see if the acid that enters the bottom of the esophagus moves to the top of the esophagus.

- Upper GI Endoscopy: If a person complains of difficulty swallowing, this procedure can show any scars or abnormal growths in the esophagus. Your doctor can then biopsy any abnormality found. This test will also show if there is any inflammation of the esophagus caused by refluxed acid.

## Treatment

If your doctor suspects silent reflux, they may prescribe reflux medication. If the medication eases your symptoms, you may be able to continue taking that medication. The medicine will also help stop any damage the silent reflux is causing. But it will not reverse it.

The most common medications used to treat silent reflux include:

- antacids
- proton pump inhibitors (PPIs)
- H2 blockers

These medicines either reduce stomach acid or prevent your stomach from creating as much stomach acid.

In addition to medicine, your doctor may recommend several lifestyle changes. These lifestyle changes are designed to help reduce risk factors that increase your chances of reflux. These lifestyle changes include:

- Stop eating and drinking at least three hours before you're planning to go to sleep.
- Prop your head up higher when you sleep.
- Identify and limit or eliminate trigger foods. These typically include chocolate, spicy foods, citrus, fried foods, and tomato-based foods.
- If you smoke, quit. Your doctor can help you find a smoking cessation program.
- Rarely, surgery is needed. But your doctor may suggest it to strengthen your esophageal sphincter.

Treatment for LPR is generally the same as that for GERD. There are four treatments for LPR:[3]

- Lifestyle changes: Quitting smoking, limiting alcohol, avoiding trigger foods, managing stress, and maintaining a weight that is healthy for you can reduce, and sometimes prevent, acid reflux.
- Diet modifications: You may want to pay attention to which foods tend to trigger your symptoms. Some common foods people need to avoid include citrus, tomatoes, spicy foods, greasy foods, coffee, and alcohol.
- Medications: Some drugs can reduce stomach acid or promote normal function. These can include proton pump inhibitors (PPIs), Histamine Receptor Antagonists, and over-the-counter (OTC) remedies like antacids.
- Surgery to prevent reflux: The most common surgery for reflux is called the Nissen fundoplication. During this procedure, a surgeon wraps part of the stomach around the lower esophageal sphincter and sews it in place.

## Complications

The thin tissue that lines your esophagus is sensitive, and stomach acid is irritating. It can burn and damage the tissue inside your esophagus, throat, and voice box. For adults, the most common complications of silent reflux include long-term irritation, tissue scarring, ulcers, and increased risk for certain cancers.

If not treated properly in children and infants, silent reflux can cause:

- breathing problems
- frequent coughing
- wheezing
- hoarseness
- difficulty swallowing
- frequent spitting up

- breathing disorders, such as apnea, or pauses in breathing

In rare cases, silent reflux may also cause growth issues. If you suspect your child has LDR, or if they've been diagnosed with it, it's important for them to receive treatment to avoid these complications.

# Which foods should I eat or avoid if I have silent reflux?

Silent reflux is also known as laryngopharyngeal reflux. It occurs when stomach acid enters the esophagus and travels up to the larynx.

Laryngopharyngeal reflux can cause no symptoms at all. For example, a person may not experience the heartburn that can come with acid reflux. This is why people call it silent reflux.

However, some people may experience symptoms such as:

- a bitter taste in the throat
- a persistent cough
- difficulty swallowing

If a person has acid reflux, they might be experiencing symptoms of gastroesophageal reflux disease (GERD).

Treating silent reflux may include trying medical treatments and making dietary changes to help prevent excessive stomach acid.

This book discusses some of the best foods to eat, some foods to avoid, and some more information about dealing with silent reflux.

**Foods to eat**

Modifying the diet can help improve silent reflux.

One 2020 study found that people with silent reflux who eat a diet that is low in protein but high in sugary, acidic, and fatty foods experience more episodes of reflux than people who adjust their diet to increase their intake of protein.

Some foods high in protein include:

- eggs
- nuts
- seeds
- fish

Some foods low in acid include:

- fresh coconuts
- lean meat
- ginger
- oatmeal
- egg whites

**To follow a diet low in sugar, a person can:**

- Read the labels of food products and avoid foods containing any type of sugar or corn syrup.
- Choose brown bread or rice over white variants, as these contain simple carbohydrates.
- Opt for whole foods, such as whole grains, fish, and nuts.

**To follow a diet low in fat, a person can:**

- Opt for fat-free or low fat dairy products.
- Opt for wholegrain foods.
- Fill up on fruits, vegetables, or sources of lean protein.

**Drinks**

Medical experts recommend that people with silent reflux drink water or herbal teas.

**Plant-based diet**

Eating a plant-based diet means avoiding all or most foods that contain animal products. Some foods that people can eat while following this diet include vegetables, fruits, whole grains, and nuts.

A 2017 study involved 184 participants. Of these participants, 99 followed a plant-based, Mediterranean-style diet consisting of the above foods, and they used standard treatment for silent reflux for 6 weeks. They also drank alkaline water.

For the same amount of time, the remaining 85 participants used the same standard treatment for silent reflux, as well as proton pump inhibitors (PPI).

At the end of the study, all of the participants experienced fewer symptoms to a similar degree.

The study concluded that following a plant-based, Mediterranean-style diet with alkaline water helped reduce symptoms just as much as taking standard medications.

This could save money, eliminate the risk of side effects, and provide a person with the other health benefits associated with following a plant-based diet.

**Foods to avoid**

Several foods may aggravate a person's silent reflux symptoms.

A person may wish to avoid the following items:

- alcohol
- chocolates
- caffeine
- peppermints

They may also wish to avoid carbonated beverages such as soda and beer, as these can weaken the lower sphincter that holds stomach acid back.

Also, acidic foods can cause stomach acid to rise into the throat. These include:

- tomatoes
- kiwis

- pineapples
- spicy foods

Some foods can irritate the lining of the esophagus. These include fried or fatty foods, such as:

- fries
- chocolate
- pastries
- cheese

Also, spicy deli meats and hot spices — including mustard, curry, and hot peppers — can directly irritate the throat lining.

**Eating habits**

As well as a person changing the food they eat, they can also make adjustments to the way they eat and live to reduce silent reflux.

For example, a person with silent reflux may wish to:

- Avoid bending over within 2 hours of eating.
- Eat smaller meals throughout the day instead of three big meals.
- Avoid lying down within 3 hours of eating.
- Avoid eating or drinking anything before going to bed.
- Inserting a 4-inch wedge under the bed to elevate the head when sleeping.

**Recipe ideas**

There are several potential ways to include generally healthy foods in small meals throughout the day.

**Breakfast**

For breakfast, a person may wish to consider eating oatmeal or another wholegrain cereal. Wholegrain cereals can be filling, which means that a person will need less to feel full until lunch.

People can add non-citric fruits such as coconut flakes to their oatmeal for added flavor.

**Lunch**

For lunch, a person may wish to consider a grilled chicken breast salad. The grilled chicken breast provides lean protein that can be filling.

**Snacks**

Eating snacks can help a person feel full throughout the day. A person can incorporate these to ensure that they are eating smaller meals throughout the day instead of only three larger meals.

A person could eat one hard-boiled egg or a piece of nonacidic fruit, such as melon.

Crackers and hummus may also satisfy hunger without causing additional stomach acid to form.

## Dinner

A person could eat a grilled fish fillet with steamed vegetables, such as broccoli, for a filling meal that should not aggravate silent reflux.

When planning dinners, a person should try to include a variety of healthy foods, such as protein sources, whole grains, vegetables, and fruits.

## Dessert

For dessert, a person can choose foods such as:

- fruit ices
- nonacidic fruits
- gelatin products
- Other at-home remedies

According to medical professionals, a person with silent reflux can also try:

- not smoking or using tobacco
- not wearing clothing that is too tight
- lying on the left side instead of the right
- chewing gum containing bicarbonate of soda
- maintaining a moderate weight
- taking any prescribed medication as a doctor instructs

**Medications**

There are several medications that may help with silent reflux.

A person should talk with a doctor about potential medications and follow their doctor's recommendations.

Some common prescription and over-the-counter medications for silent reflux include:

- PPIs: These are the most effective treatment option. A person can expect fewer symptoms after 4–6 weeks of taking this medication as prescribed.
- H2 blockers: These are antihistamines and can be especially effective at night.
- Antacids: These medications may be available over the counter or with a prescription.
- Medications and dosages may differ for people with GERD. For example, a person with silent reflux may require a higher dosage of a medication for a longer period of time.

## Natural and home remedies

**1. Quitting smoking**

Smoking has a negative effect on health. However, people may be unaware that smoke, even secondhand smoke, can increase acid reflux.

The lower esophageal sphincter (LES) is the valve between the esophagus, or food pipe, and stomach. The LES stops stomach acid from flowing back up into the esophagus.

According to a 2015 review, smoking reduces the pressure on the LES, making acid reflux possible. Quitting smoking should normalize this pressure, reducing the likelihood of acid reflux.

2. **Using calming techniques**

   Focusing on the discomfort that acid reflux causes can lead to anxiety and worsen how a person feels.

   Individuals experiencing anxiety can try box breathing techniques to manage the rapid breathing and dizziness that can occur with anxiety.

   Although staying calm will not stop acid reflux, it can help a person avoid experiencing more severe symptoms.

3. **Avoiding trigger substances**

   People may find that certain foods and drinks can trigger acid reflux. This can be due to items increasing stomach acid production or reducing the LES's ability to stop acid from flowing into the esophagus.

Eliminating these trigger items from the diet may help people reduce the frequency or severity of their acid reflux symptoms.

**Common trigger substances include:**

- coffee
- alcohol
- mint
- tomato
- fatty foods
- spicy foods

## 4. Adding ginger into the diet

Some research suggests that ginger may help with nausea, vomiting, and other symptoms. However, the limited quality of included evidence means that more research is necessary to confirm these benefits.

Based on the existing evidence, researchers suggest a daily dose of 1,500 milligrams of ginger. It is possible that a higher intake could have adverse effects.

Ginger is an easy ingredient to incorporate into the diet. People can try:

- adding it to hot water to make ginger tea
- including it in a stir-fry
- boiling it in a soup
- grating it raw onto salads or cereals

Individuals who dislike the taste of ginger can mask it by including ginger in recipes with other strong flavors.

5. **Maintaining a moderate weight**

Eating a balanced diet is key for a person's general health, and it can also help them manage their body weight.

According to Dietary Guidelines for Americans 2020 – 2025, approximately 74% of all adults in the U.S. have overweight or obesity.

Research suggests that there is a link between having obesity and an increased risk of developing acid reflux.

The reason for the link seems to be that excess fat around the abdominal area puts pressure on the stomach, making the body work harder to keep acid down.

People with obesity may find that reaching and maintaining a moderate weight helps them reduce the frequency of acid reflux.

It is important that people focus on safe ways to lose weight, as losing too much weight too quickly may cause health problems.

6. **Chewing sugar-free gum after meals**

An older study from 2005 suggests that chewing gum can increase swallowing frequency, improving the clearance rate of reflux in the esophagus. However, there is no follow-up evidence to support this claim.

Chewing also boosts saliva production, which can help weaken stomach acid.

However, it is important to avoid chewing gums containing sugar, which may make the symptoms worse or cause dental erosion.

People with acid reflux should also avoid mint-flavored gums, such as peppermint and spearmint, as these may also aggravate symptoms.

## 7. Trying herbal tea

Some drinks, including coffee and alcohol, may increase the symptoms of acid reflux. Replacing these beverages with decaffeinated herbal teas may help reduce the likelihood of acid reflux occurring.

Herbal teas can also help improve digestion and ease symptoms such as dizziness or nausea.

Popular herbal teas include:

- chamomile tea
- licorice tea
- green tea
- fennel tea
- fruit teas

It is best to avoid mint teas, as they may trigger acid reflux.

## 8. Adding high fiber foods into the diet

Fiber is an important part of a balanced diet. It can help a person feel full and aid digestion, easing the symptoms of acid reflux.

Fiber rich foods that a person can start introducing into their diet include:

- whole-wheat breakfast cereals
- porridge oats
- granary bread
- 100% whole-wheat pasta
- bulgur wheat
- brown rice
- potato skin — for example, on baked potatoes

- beans
- lentils
- garbanzo beans
- broccoli

9. **Keeping a food diary**

Keeping a diary and tracking when acid reflux occurs can help a person feel more in control of their body.

In addition to their symptoms, they can note the foods that they have eaten and any changes to their behaviors or habits. This approach can help a person identify any acid reflux triggers, which they can then avoid where possible to prevent acid reflux from recurring.

If someone is unable to identify and eliminate factors that cause or worsen acid reflux or if they have concerns about their symptoms, they should contact a doctor. They may have GERD or another health condition. A doctor can diagnose the issue and help them devise a treatment plan.

Recipes for LPR

## 1. Spaghetti Squash Pad Thai With Tempeh

**Ingredients**

- 1 | small spaghetti squash (about 1.5-2 lbs)
- 7 oz | tempeh, sliced into thin strips
- 2 | large carrots, cut julienne style
- 1 1/2 cup | green beans, chopped into inch pieces
- 2 | eggs
- 3 tbsp | dry roasted almonds, loosely chopped
- 1 tbsp | sesame oil
- 1 tbsp | extra virgin olive oil
- 1 tbsp | soy sauce
- Cilantro to garnish
- Sesame seeds to garnish

**Sauce**

- 1/3 cup | soy sauce
- 3 tbsp | fish sauce
- 3 tbsp | brown sugar
- 1 tbsp | sesame oil
- 1 tbsp | fresh ginger, grated
- Zest from 2 limes

**Directions**

- Preheat oven to 375 degrees Fahrenheit. Cut spaghetti squash in half lengthwise and remove seeds. Place face down on a silicone baking mat or parchment paper and bake for 45 minutes.
- When the squash is done, use a fork to remove it from the shell and set aside until ready to use.
- While the squash is cooking start making the sauce. Combine all the ingredients that are under sauce, into a small saucepan and mix well until sugar is dissolved. Then heat the pan over

a medium heat, cook for about 5 minutes, stirring frequently until the sauce becomes thicker, then set aside.
- Now time to lightly fry the tempeh. In a large skillet over medium heat add 1 tbsp of sesame oil, and 1 tbsp of olive oil, along with 1 tbsp of soy sauce. Add the tempeh cooking on each side for about 4 minutes. It should be getting slightly brown on each side. Once the tempeh is cooked remove from the pan.
- Using the same skillet start sautéing the vegetables. Add the carrots and green beans and cook until they begin to soften, about 8-10 minutes. Push the veggies to one side, and then add the eggs to the other side and scramble them
- Now add the tempeh back to the pan and the shredded spaghetti squash and sauce. Mix well,

but carefully so that you don't break up the tempeh too much.
- Add salt to taste if needed and garnish with the almonds, sesame seeds and cilantro!

2. **Miso Ginger Chicken**

**Ingredients**
- 1 lb | chicken breast, cubed
- 1 | shallot, diced (optional)
- 2 1/2 tbsp | soy sauce
- 1 tbsp | fresh ginger, minced
- 1 1/2 tsp | white miso paste
- 1 tbsp | sesame oil
- 2 tsp | cornstartch
- 1/4 tsp | asafetida
- 1 tbsp | extra virgin olive oil
- Sesame seeds to garnish

**Directions**

- In a skillet over medium heat add the olive oil and allow it to heat up. Once the oil is hot add in the shallot and cook until it begins to soften. Then add the chicken to the skillet. Make sure to flip occasionally, it should take between 7-10 minutes to cook through.
- While the chicken is cooking, start working on the sauce. In a small bowl mix together the soy sauce, ginger, miso paste, sesame oil, asafetida, and cornstarch. Mix well so there are no clumps of miso or cornstarch, a whisk works best for this.
- When the chicken is cooked add in the sauce and cook until it is thoroughly heated and has thickened, stirring occasionally, about 3-5 minutes.
- Garnish with sesame seeds and serve with veggies and your favorite grain!

### 3. Tomato-Free Rice And Bean Bake

**Ingredients**

- 2 cups | uncooked regular long-grain white rice
- cups | chicken or vegetable broth
- 2 | 15 oz. cans of beans of your choice, undrained!
- 1 | shallot, diced
- 1 1/2 tbsp | cumin
- 2 tsp | dried oregano
- 1 tbsp | paprika
- 1/4 tsp | asafetida
- 1/2 tbsp | salt
- 3/4 cup | cheddar cheese, shredded
- Cilantro (if desired)

**Directions**

- Preheat oven to 350 degrees Fahrenheit. In a dutch oven or a casserole dish (ungreased) mix all the ingredients together, and then cover with a lid.
- Bake for one hour, or until all liquid is absorbed. Take out of the oven and sprinkle cheese on top, and cover again until cheese is nice and melted, about 2-3 minutes.
- Top with cilantro if desired, and enjoy!

4. **Pasta With Collard Greens And Lemon Zest**

**Ingredients**

- 1 | bunch of collard green leaves, about 10-12 leaves
- 8 oz | spaghetti pasta
- 2 tbsp | olive oil
- 4 tbsp | pine nuts

- 1 tbsp | ginger, grated or chopped finely
- Zest from 2 lemons
- Parmesan cheese (optional)
- Salt to taste

**Directions**

- Bring a large pot of salted water to a boil and boil the spaghetti noodles. Cook and set aside
- De-stem the collard greens and chop the collards into small pieces, no more than 1/2 inch wide.
- Heat a skillet over medium heat and add the pine nuts, until they are a nice golden brown color, turning frequently. Set aside when done.
- Using the same skillet over medium heat add 1 tbsp of olive oil and the ginger to the pan. Allow the ginger to simmer until fragrant then add in the collard greens and the lemon zest.

- Cook the greens until they are mostly tender, about 5 minutes, turning frequently.
- In the pot that the noodles were cooked, or the skillet combine all the ingredients; pasta, pine nuts, and collard mixture. Add more olive oil one tsp at a time, until the pasta is nice and oiled, but not adding more than 3 tsp total.
- Salt to taste and add Parmesan on top and serve!

## 5. Broccoli And Cheddar Cheese Bites

**Ingredients**

- 5 | large eggs
- 1 cup | broccoli, chopped very small
- 1/3 cup & 6 tsp | cheddar cheese, shredded
- 1/4 tsp | dried oregano
- 1/8 tsp | salt

**Directions**

- Preheat the oven to 350 degrees Fahrenheit. Spray a muffin tin with nonstick cooking spray, or add a bit of melted coconut oil to each muffin cup and spread around.
- In a large bowl whisk all of the eggs, until well blended, then add in the cup of broccoli, oregano, salt and 1/3 cup of cheddar cheese. Mix well.
- Pour the mixture into the each of the muffin cup (or use a ladle) distributing evenly. Be careful not to overfill as it can overflow in your oven! I would also maybe recommend putting a baking sheet underneath your muffin tin, if you are worried about it.
- Bake for 23-38 minutes, or until a toothpick comes out clean. Remove from the oven, and let cool for about 5 minutes, then take a knife

around the side of each muffin and then scoop them out.

- Can be kept in the fridge for up to 6 days. Takes about 45-60 seconds to reheat in the microwave!

## 6. Thai Coconut Soup

**Ingredients**

- 1 | bag of frozen cauliflower
- 1 cup | fresh green beans, chopped into 2-3 inch pieces
- 3 | large carrots, cut into matchsticks
- 1 (8 oz) | container of mushrooms, sliced
- 1 | celeriac root, diced
- 1 | bunch of Tuscan kale, de-stemmed and cut into 1 inch pieces
- 1 | shallot, diced
- 1 tbsp | coconut oil

- 2 1/2 tbsp | "Curry" spice mix
- 1 tbsp | fresh ginger, grated
- 1/2 tsp | asafetida
- 2 (14 oz) | full fat coconut milk
- 4 cups | vegetable broth
- Salt to taste
- Cilantro to garnish

**Directions**

- Heat the coconut oil in a large dutch oven over medium heat, once the coconut oil has melted add the shallot and grated ginger, stirring often. Once onions are soft, add in the "curry" spice mix and asafetida, and cook for 2 more minutes.
- Add in the 4 cups of vegetable broth, the 2 cans of coconut milk, mushrooms, green beans, carrots, and celeriac root. Bring to a simmer and cook for 12-15 minutes, until the vegetables are just starting to get tender.

- Now add in the bag of frozen cauliflower and cook until the cauliflower is heated through.
- Once the cauliflower is heated through, add the tuscan kale and cook for about 2 minutes, until slightly wilted.
- Salt to taste and serve! Top with cilantro if desired.

7. **Vegetarian Sausage with Braised Cabbage**

**Ingredients**
- 1 head fresh green cabbage, thinly sliced
- 1 link Vegetarian Sausage, such as Tofurky Italian Sausage or Boca Italian Sausage, sliced
- 1 tablespoon Olive Oil
- 2 tablespoons of water
- Optional salt, pepper, and a seasoning blend such as Mrs. Dash.

**Directions**

- Chop the Cabbage into thin strips
- Slice the Vegetarian Sausage into rounds
- Saute both in the Olive Oil and water.
- Cover and cook for about 10 minutes over low heat, stirring every so often, until the cabbage is soft & lightly browned.
- Season to taste with salt, pepper, and a seasoning blend

8. **Banana Ginger Energy Smoothie**

**Ingredients**

- 1/2 cup ice
- 2 cups milk
- 2 ripe bananas
- 1 cup yogurt
- 1/2 tsp fresh ginger (peeled and grated fine)
- 2 tbsp brown sugar or honey (optional)

- In a blender, add the ice, milk, yogurt, bananas, and ginger. Blend until smooth. Add sugar as needed.

9. **Mushroom Stock**

**Ingredients**
- 1 t canola oil
- 2 leeks, white and light green parts only, sliced
- 3.5 ounces shiitake mushrooms, chopped
- 8 ounces baby portabella mushrooms, chopped
- 3 medium carrots, grated
- 1 tablespoon white wine, tomato juice, or lemon juice
- 2 garlic cloves or 1 teaspoon grated ginger
- 1/2 teaspoon black peppercorns
- 3 sprigs fresh thyme
- 4 parsley stems
- 9 cups cold water

**Directions**

- Place a large saucepan over moderate heat. Add the oil to the hot pan, then add the leeks to the hot oil and sweat for 3 minutes. Add the mushrooms and sweat for 2 minutes. Add the carrots and cook until the vegetables are tender. Add your acid of choice (wine, lemon juice or tomato juice) to deglaze the pan. Stir in the acid with a wooden spoon, scraping the bottom to lift up any "fond" (crust) on the bottom of the pan.
- Add the remaining ingredients. Bring to a boil and reduce to a simmer for 40 minutes. Cool slightly and strain through a fine-mesh strainer. Cool completely if freezing.
- Makes 6 cups, 1/2 cup per serving

## 10. Calm Carrot Salad for Acid Reflux

### Ingredients

- 2 tbsp Brown sugar
- 2 tsp Olive oil
- 1/4 tsp salt
- 1 tsp Dried oregano
- 2 tbsp Orange juice
- 1/4 lb mesclun greens
- 2 tbsp Raisins
- 1 lb carrots ; peeled, trimmed, and grated

### Instructions

- Step 1: Take a mixing bowl, mix the raisins, orange juice, brown sugar, olive oil, oregano, and salt together. Let sit for about 5 minutes.
- Step 2. Pour your dressing over the carrots and mix very patiently and thoroughly so they're mixed together evenly.

- Step 3. Season with additional salt as per your dietary desires.
- Step 4. Serve over mesclun leaves and take a trip to cuisine enjoyment!

## 11. Cantaloupe Gazpacho

**Ingredients**
- 1 medium cantaloupe (peeled, seeded, chopped)
- 1 small cucumber (peeled, chopped)
- 2 tablespoons chopped red onion
- 2 teaspoons kosher salt
- 1/2 cup extra virgin olive oil
- Kosher salt and freshly ground black pepper
- Thinly sliced fresh mint
- Purée 1 medium cantaloupe (peeled, seeded, chopped), 1 small cucumber (peeled, chopped), 2 tablespoons chopped red onion, 2 teaspoons

kosher salt, and 1/3 cup water in a blender until smooth. With motor running, drizzle in 1/2 cup extra-virgin olive oil; season with kosher salt and freshly ground black pepper. Serve gazpacho chilled, topped with thinly sliced fresh mint.
- Start Cooking

## 12. Orange Thyme Chicken

**Ingredients**
- 3 Tbsp orange marmalade
- 2 tsp white wine vinegar
- 1/8 tsp salt
- 1 tsp fresh thyme leaves
- fresh ground black pepper (to taste)
- 8 ounces boneless skinless chicken breast
- 2 tsp olive oil
- 1/4 cup white wine
- 1 tsp unsalted butter

**Instructions**

- Place a medium skillet in the oven and preheat the oven to 325F.
- Place the marmalade, vinegar, salt, thyme, and pepper in a small bowl and whisk together.
- Add the chicken to the bowl and toss to coat well.
- Place the olive oil in the skillet and add the chicken, then place in the oven. (There will be some leftover marinade; reserve the remaining marinade.)
- Roast the chicken for approximately 10 minutes, then turn the chicken over and top with the remaining marinade, then return to the oven.
- Roast for an additional 7-10 minutes, or until the chicken reaches 160F.
- Remove the chicken from the oven and place on a cutting board to rest.

- Place the skillet on the range over medium-high heat and add the white wine to deglaze the pan. Stir frequently and scrape up any bits that may be sticking to the pan.
- Simmer and reduce the liquid by about 1/2, then add the butter and remove from heat. Whisk the butter into the sauce until the butter melts, then serve on top of the chicken.

13. Chicken cutlets with sauteed mushrooms

**Ingredients**
- 1 pound boneless, skinless chicken breasts (or chicken breast cutlets)
- 1/3 cup whole wheat flour
- 2 tablespoons olive oil
- 3 tablespoons butter
- 2 cups mushrooms, sliced

- 1/3 cup white wine (or low sodium chicken broth)
- Salt and pepper to taste

**Directions**

- Slice the chicken breasts in half crosswise, so you have thin pieces of chicken, and trim any excess fat. (Skip this step if you're using cutlets.)
- Season the chicken with salt and pepper.
- Place the flour in a bowl, and dredge the chicken in the flour until it is lightly coated.
- Heat the oil in a large skillet over medium high heat.
- Add the chicken to the skillet and brown on both sides, 3-4 minutes per side.
- When the chicken is done, remove it from the pan and set it aside.
- Turn the heat down to medium. Add the butter and mushrooms to the same pan and sauté until the mushrooms are soft (about 5 minutes).

- When the mushrooms are done, add the wine or chicken broth to deglaze the pan and stir well.
- Add the chicken back to the pan and cook until sauce has thickened (about 2 minutes).

14. **Greek pasta**

**Ingredients**
- 8 oz. whole wheat penne pasta
- 8 ounces boneless, skinless chicken, chopped
- 16 calamata olives
- 1 cup reduced fat feta cheese crumbles
- 3 cloves garlic, minced
- 1.5 cup whole mushrooms
- 1 cup cherry tomatoes, halved
- 1 tbsp balsamic vinegar

**Directions**

- Cook pasta. In a separate pan, cook chicken and garlic in balsamic vinegar. When chicken is cooked thoroughly, add mushrooms and tomatoes to heat.
- Mix cooked pasta, chicken, garlic and mushrooms. Add olices and top with feta crumbles.
- This meal could easily become vegetarian by omitting chicken. Add onion or peppers for a twist.

15. **Healthy Pasta Primavera Recipe**

**Ingredients**

- 8 ounces whole wheat pasta such as penne
- 2 cups of warm prepared marinara sauce look for a low-fat, low-sugar variety
- 2 teaspoons olive oil

- 1 cup of small broccoli florets
- 1/2 cup of peeled carrots cut into 1/4 inch pieces
- 1 yellow squash halved and thinly sliced
- 1 cup of mushrooms thinly sliced
- 1/2 cup chopped onion
- 2 teaspoons minced garlic
- salt and pepper to taste
- 1/2 cup freshly grated parmesan cheese
- Optional: 2 tablespoons chopped parsley.

**Instructions**

- Cook the pasta in salted water according to package instructions.
- While the pasta is cooking, heat the olive oil in a large pan over medium-high heat.
- Add the onions to the pan and cook for 3-4 minutes, or until they've started to soften.

- Add the broccoli, carrots, squash, and mushrooms to the pan. Season the vegetables with salt and pepper to taste.
- Add 2 tablespoons of water to the pan. Cook for 5-7 minutes or until vegetables are tender and starting to brown.
- Stir in the garlic and cook for 30 seconds more.
- Add the cooked pasta and marinara sauce in the pan; toss to coat.
- Sprinkle with parmesan cheese and serve. Top with chopped parsley if desired.

**Notes**

- Nutritional facts:
- Please keep in mind that the nutritional information is calculated using a nutrition facts calculator. It is a rough estimate and can vary greatly based on products used.

## 16. Banana Ginger Energy

Meals that are low in fat and acid, but high in whole grains, vegetables, and certain fruits can help you avoid heartburn.

In , authors Jamie Koufman, MD, Jordan Stern, MD, and French master chef Marc Bauer offer healthy recipes that fit the bill.

**Ingredients**
- ½ cup ice
- 2 cups milk
- 2 bananas, ripe
- 1 cup yogurt
- ½ tsp. fresh ginger, peeled and grated fine
- 2 tbsp. brown sugar or honey (optional)

### Directions

- In a blender, add the ice, milk, yogurt, bananas, and ginger.
- Blend until smooth.
- Add sugar as needed.

### 17. Gala Apple Honeydew Smoothie

### Ingredients

- 2 cups honeydew melon (peeled, seeded, cut into chunks)
- 4 tbsp. fresh , skin removed
- 1 Gala apple (peeled, cored, cut in half)
- 1/16 tsp. lime zest (use a grater to get the zest)
- 1 ½ cups ice
- ¼ tsp. salt

**Directions**

- In a blender, add the melon, ice, aloe vera, apple, salt, and lime zest.
- Begin blending on Pulse before switching to High. Stop and stir the mixture as needed to get a smooth consistency.

18. **Museli-Style-Oatmeal**

**Ingredients**

- 1 cup instant oatmeal
- 1 cup milk
- 2 tbsp. raisins (brought to a boil, drained)
- ½ banana, diced
- ½ golden apple, peeled, diced
- Pinch of salt
- 2 tsp. sugar or honey

**Directions**

- The evening before (or at least 2 hours before), mix the oatmeal, milk, raisins, salt, and sugar (or honey) together in a bowl.
- Cover and place in the refrigerator.
- Add fruit before serving.
- If the mix is too thick, add milk.

## 19. Instant Polenta With Sesame Seeds

**Ingredients**

- ¾ cup instant polenta or corn meal
- 3 cups whole milk
- 3 tbsp. brown sugar
- 1 tsp. orange extract
- ½ tsp. vanilla extract
- Salt to taste
- 1 tbsp. sesame seeds

**Directions**

- Bring the milk to a boil.
- Add the polenta or corn meal and whisk vigorously to prevent lumps.
- Cook until creamy.
- Add the sugar, salt, and vanilla, and orange extract just before serving.
- Serve in a bowl and sprinkle with sesame seeds.

20. **Calm Carrot Salad**

**Ingredients**

- 1 lb. carrots (peeled, trimmed, and grated)
- ¼ lb. mesclun greens
- 2 tbsp. raisins
- 2 tbsp. orange juice
- 1 tsp. dried oregano
- 2 tbsp. brown sugar
- 2 tsp. olive oil

- ¼ tsp. salt

**Directions**

- In a bowl, mix the raisins, orange juice, oregano, brown sugar, olive oil, and salt. Let sit for about 5 minutes.
- Pour the dressing over the carrots and mix thoroughly.
- Season with additional salt, as needed.
- Serve over mesclun leaves.

## 21. Black Bean Cilantro

**Ingredients**

- 8 oz. canned black beans
- 1 pint chicken stock
- ½ cup fresh cilantro
- Salt to taste
- 1 tbsp. nonfat sour cream

- Directions
- Bring the chicken stock to a boil. Add the beans, cilantro, and salt.
- Cook 30 minutes on low heat.
- Blend with a hand blender to the desired consistency.
- Season, as needed.
- Serve in a soup bowl and garnish with 1 tsp. nonfat sour cream and a sprig of cilantro

## 22. Fresh Young Coconut and Banana Smoothie

Coconut and banana make a delightful combination in smoothies. Together they are good source of magnesium, potassium and fiber. As well as many different vitamins and minerals.

**Ingredients**

- 1 ½ cups – fresh coconut water
- 1 cup – fresh, coconut meat, chopped
- 1 – 2 bananas, chopped and frozen
- ¼ cup almond milk(optional)
- 4-5 ice cubes

**Instructions**

- Add all ingredients in a blender and blend till it reaches a consistency you desire.
- Add a little coconut water, or almond milk if the smoothie is too thick.

## 23. Parsley Smoothie

This smoothie will not only provide relief from acid reflux but it can also give you energy and refreshment on a hot, summer day. This refreshing and energizing smoothie is a nice blend of parsley, mango, pear and coconut.

**Ingredients**
- ½ bunch -parsley with stems cut
- 2 small pears – cored
- 1 coconut – meat and water
- ¾ cup mango – peeled

**Instructions**
- Add coconut water to a blender. Then throw in coconut, pear and mango.
- Finally, add the greens and blend on high speed for 30 seconds to a minute until creamy.

## 24. Strawberry Watermelon Smoothie

Both watermelon and certain berries can be great for treating acid reflux. This combination is delicious and truly delightful. It is rich in fiber and can help revitalize you.

**Ingredients**
- 9 cups – watermelon, cut into pieces and with seeds removed
- 12 ounces – frozen strawberries
- ¼ cup – freshly squeezed lemon juice

**Instructions**
- First, take the watermelon pieces in a blender and blend for 30 seconds.
- Now add the strawberries and lemon juice then blend until smooth.
- Serve immediately, or refrigerate for later.

## 25. Banana Ginger Smoothie

Keep those heartburn and GERD symptoms away with this smoothie. Banana is an alkaline fruit which can neutralize the acid in your body. Ginger has anti-inflammatory properties and it can provide relief from heartburn and other stomach ailments.

You can also add honey to help sweeten this smoothie. Honey is rich in probiotics and it can quell acid reflux.

**Ingredients**
- 2 cups – low-fat milk
- 2 small bananas – ripe
- 1 cup yoghurt – unsweetened
- 1 tsp ginger – peeled and grated
- 1 tbsp – honey

- ½ cup – ice

**Instructions**

- Peel your bananas and roughly chop them. Add them into the blender.
- Add milk, yogurt, ginger, ice and blend until smooth.
- Add a tablespoon of honey and blend for a few seconds.
- Enjoy!

## 26. Pineapple Yogurt Smoothie

The combination of ingredients in this smoothie can help reduce your acid reflux. Plus, it is absolutely tasty!

**Ingredients**

- 1 ½ cups – pineapple, chopped

- 1 banana
- ½ cup pineapple juice or water
- ½ cup – greek yoghurt
- ½ cup – ice

**Instructions**
- Put all the ingredients in a blender
- Blend until it reaches a nice, drinkable consistency

## 27. Apple Honeydew Smoothie

Get your sweet tooth craving and get rid of acid reflux symptoms with this versatile smoothie. The apple and honeydew melon work together to give you a smoothie that is better than most.

**Ingredients**

- 2 cups – honeydew melon, peeled, seeded and cut into chunks
- 4 tbsp – fresh aloe vera, skin removed
- 1 gala apple – peeled, cored and cut in half
- 1/16 tsp. lime zest
- 1 ½ cups – ice
- ¼ tsp – salt, to taste

**Instructions**

- Add melon, apple, aloe vera, lime zest (after grating it) and salt in a blender.
- Pulse the ingredients in a blender for a few seconds. Then blend on high.
- Stir the mixture until smooth.

## 28. Carrot Banana Smoothie

Carrots are rich in Vitamin A, which is good for vision and skin. Bananas are a natural antacid and it can provide relief from heartburn and reflux.

**Ingredients**
- 2 carrots
- 1 banana
- ½ cup almond milk, unsweetened
- A pinch of cinnamon
- A pinch of nutmeg
- A handful of chia seeds
- 2 tbsp coconut cream
- 1 clove
- 2 dates

## Instructions

- Blend almond milk, banana, spices, dates and coconut cream until smooth.
- Add the chopped carrots then blend everything until smooth and frothy.
- Finally, garnish by sprinkling chia seeds.

## 29. Green Smoothie

Green smoothies are very soothing when you have tummy problems. They are super healthy and can provide relief from acid reflux and GERD symptoms.

## Ingredients

- 1/2 Head each of kale and spinach
- 1 Mango
- 1 Apple
- 1 cup – fresh strawberries

- 1 cup – greek or plain yogurt
- Honey, to taste

**Instructions**

- Add all the ingredients in a blender and blend until smooth.
- Now add honey to help sweeten the smoothie.
- Add several ice cubes and blend to thicken the smoothie.

## 30. Beetroot and Carrot Smoothie

Alkalizing vegetables like beetroot, carrot, celery and ginger combine beautifully in this super smoothie to help battle stomach acids. Even though this smoothie is vegetable rich, it has notes of sweetness which makes it easy to savor.

**Ingredients**
- 1 small beet – peeled and cut into chunks
- 1 red apple – cored and cut into chunks
- 1cup – carrot juice
- 1 stalk of celery – cut into chunks
- 1 cup – unsweetened almond milk
- ½-inch fresh ginger – peeled

**Instructions**
- Blend all ingredients in a blender until smooth.

- Carrots and beets will take a long time to blend, so blend on high for 2-3 minutes.

## 31. Vegetable Anti-Heartburn Smoothie

This wonderful and healthy, anti-heartburn smoothie can work wonders against acid reflux. It is also extremely healthy and refreshing.

**Ingredients**
- A handful of – raw spinach (regular or baby spinach)
- 3 to 4 – uncooked broccoli florets
- 1 leaf of kale – fresh and without stems
- ½ of a cucumber
- 3 or 4-inch piece horseradish or a handful of regular radishes, chopped Water as needed
- ½ peeled orange to sweeten, optional

**Instructions**

- Combine everything in a blender.
- Blend until completely smooth. Add water if needed.
- Once the desired texture is reached, stop, pour into a glass and enjoy!

## Conclusion

Diagnosing and treating reflux is the key to preventing symptoms and avoiding damage to your esophagus, throat, lungs, and voice box. A diagnosis is often quite painless and easy.

Treatment may be even more painless. Most people will take a daily medication and make several lifestyle changes. With these lifestyle changes, you may find the medication unnecessary.

LPR is a form of acid reflux that occurs when the upper esophageal sphincter malfunctions, causing acid to pool in the throat. You may experience symptoms like coughing, throat clearing, sore throat, hoarseness, and weak voice when this happens.

Often people find that certain foods trigger their symptoms. So, to manage symptoms, you may need to modify your diet. In addition, OTC and prescription medications can reduce or prevent symptoms. In more extreme situations, surgery is also an option.

Silent reflux occurs when stomach acid travels into the esophagus and up to the larynx, causing discomfort and symptoms such as a persistent cough and a bitter taste in the throat.

There are several foods that can help reduce the acid in the stomach, dilute this acid, or keep a person feeling fuller with less food.

A person should avoid eating foods that aggravate their condition, including spicy foods, fatty foods, and foods with high acidity levels.

A person can make several lifestyle changes and work with a doctor to take appropriate medication to help treat their silent reflux.

Made in the USA
Monee, IL
12 May 2022